I0223137

104 Diabetes Meal and Juice Recipes:

Control Your Condition Naturally Using Nutrient-Rich Ingredients

By

Joe Correa CSN

COPYRIGHT

© 2017 Live Stronger Faster Inc.

All rights reserved

Reproduction or translation of any part of this work beyond that permitted by section 107 or 108 of the 1976 United States Copyright Act without the permission of the copyright owner is unlawful.

This publication is designed to provide accurate and authoritative information in regard to the subject matter covered. It is sold with the understanding that neither the author nor the publisher is engaged in rendering medical advice. If medical advice or assistance is needed, consult with a doctor. This book is considered a guide and should not be used in any way detrimental to your health. Consult with a physician before starting this nutritional plan to make sure it's right for you.

ACKNOWLEDGEMENTS

This book is dedicated to all the people in the world that have mild or serious illnesses so that you may find a solution and make the necessary changes in your life.

104 Diabetes Meal and Juice Recipes:

Control Your Condition Naturally Using Nutrient-Rich Ingredients

By

Joe Correa CSN

CONTENTS

ABOUT THE AUTHOR

After years of Research, I honestly believe in the positive effects that proper nutrition can have over the body and mind. My knowledge and experience has helped me live healthier throughout the years and which I have shared with family and friends. The more you know about eating and drinking healthier, the sooner you will want to change your life and eating habits.

Nutrition is a key part in the process of being healthy and living longer so get started today. The first step is the most important and the most significant.

INTRODUCTION

104 Diabetes Meal and Juice Recipes: Control Your Condition Naturally Using Nutrient-Rich Ingredients

By Joe Correa CSN

Physicians diagnose diabetes when a patient is suffering from an unexplained history of illness or abdominal pain that lasts for a couple of weeks. If you're diagnosed with diabetes, you will be referred to a specialist for this disease. The specific treatment of diabetes means that the majority of medical care is run by hospitals, rather than the family doctors. However, at the end of a day, you're left with your disease and it is up to you to maintain a healthy diet after that.

The main symptoms are the same for both – kids and adults. Usually, these symptoms occur within a few weeks and include thirst, weight loss, fatigue, frequent urination, etc. Symptoms that are more specific to children are bellyaches, headaches, or behavior problems.

In this book, you will find some delicious recipes and tips you can follow when cooking diabetic friendly food. To help you get started with this style of cooking, a list of recipes will be outlined for you. You simply have to follow the instructions and start your new nutritional lifestyle. The best part of all is that you don't need to be a cooking expert to achieve the desired taste and effect in the food you make. The recipes in this book are simple enough for everyone to prepare.

104 DIABETES MEAL AND JUICE RECIPES: CONTROL YOUR CONDITION NATURALLY USING NUTRIENT-RICH INGREDIENTS

MEALS

1. Kick-start Pancakes

Ingredients:

1/3 cup of all-purpose flour

½ cup of skim milk

1 tbsp of baking powder

½ tsp of salt

3 tbsp of sugar substitute blend

1 egg

2 tbsp of olive oil

Preparation:

Combine the ingredients in a bowl and mix well with a fork or an electric mixer. You want to get a nice smooth and foamy mixture. Cover and let it stand for about 10 minutes.

Heat up some oil in a frying pan. Use about ½ cup of the pancake mixture to make one pancake. Fry for about 1-2 minutes on each side and serve.

Top with warm chocolate topping, strawberries, whipped cream or any other, sugar-free topping you like.

How to prepare warm sugar-free chocolate topping?

Ingredients:

4oz unsweetened chocolate (85% cocoa)

1 cup of whipped cream

½ cup of coconut oil

8 tbsp of Agave Syrup

2 tbsp of unsweetened, raw cocoa powder

2 tsp of liquid vanilla extract

Preparation:

Heat up the coconut oil over a medium heat. Melt the chocolate and stir in agave syrup, cocoa powder, vanila extract and whipped cream. Mix well using an electric mixer.

Use to top pancakes.

Nutrition information per serving: Kcal: 312 Protein: 14.5g, Carbs: 42g, Fats: 18g, Sodium: 350mg

2.   Warm Banana Porridge

Ingredients

½ cup rolled oats

1 cup of water

1 cup of almond milk

1 banana, sliced

1 tbsp of LSA mix

Sultanas to taste

1 tbsp of manuka honey (or pure maple syrup)

1 tsp of cinnamon, ground

Preparation:

Bring one cup of water to a boiling point. Place the oats in it and cook for a couple of minutes.

Reduce the heat and add one cup of almond milk. Simmer until the oats are soft. Stir in the sliced bananas, cinnamon, honey, one teaspoon of LSA mix and sultanas to taste.

Nutrition information per serving: Kcal: 256 Protein: 31.3g, Carbs: 24g, Fats: 11g, Sodium: 154mg

3.   Mango Super Oatmeal

Ingredients:

1 pack of quick-cooking oats

½ cup chopped mango

1 tsp agave syrup or raw honey

¼ tsp of cinnamon

Preparation:

Use package directions to cook the oats.

Stir in agave syrup and cinnamon. Mix well

Top with mango and serve.

Nutrition information per serving: Kcal: 219 Protein: 14g, Carbs: 29g, Fats: 10g, Sodium: 190mg

4.   Mr. Almond and Mrs. Apple Oats

Ingredients

½ cup rolled oats

1 cup of water

1 Alkmene apple, peeled and grated

1 apple, sliced

2 tbsp of almond yogurt, sugar-free

1 tsp of cinnamon, ground

Preparation

Boil the water and add oats. Briefly cook (2-3 minutes) and reduce the heat.

Add one grated Alkmene apple and one teaspoon of cinnamon. Simmer for another ten minutes. Remove from the heat.

Top with almond yogurt and sliced apple. Serve warm.

Nutrition information per serving: Kcal: 190 Protein: 12g, Carbs: 35g, Fats: 8.9g, Sodium: 219mg

5.   Oatmeal with Almonds and Cinnamon

Ingredients:

1 pack of quick-cooking oats

¼ cup of toasted almonds, chopped

1 tsp of cinnamon

1 tsp of agave syrup

2oz sliced mango

Preparation:

Boil the water and add oats. Briefly cook (for several minutes) and reduce the heat.

Stir in cinnamon and agave syrup. Top with almonds and slices of mango.

Serve warm.

Nutrition information per serving: Kcal: 119 Protein: 17g, Carbs: 27g, Fats: 9g, Sodium: 158mg

6.   Whipped Cream Pancakes

Ingredients

½ cup of all-purpose flour

1 egg

1 cup of coconut milk, sugar-free

1cup raspberries

1 tsp of vanilla extract, sugar-free

Cooking oil

2 cups whipped cream for topping, sugar-free

Preparation:

Combine all all-purpose flour and vanilla extract in a large bowl. Gently whisk in coconut milk and one egg. Mix well with an electric mixer.

Spread some cooking oil over a small, non-stick frying pan.

Pour about ½ cup of pancake mixture and cook for about three minutes on each side

Top with one tablespoon of whipped cream and raspberries.

Nutrition information per serving: Kcal: 298 Protein: 31g, Carbs: 42g, Fats: 26g, Sodium: 335mg

7.   Wild Very Berry Smoothie

Ingredients:

1 cup of mixed berries

2 cups of skim milk

1 tsp of honey (can be replaced with agave syrup)

1 tbsp of pumpkin seeds

½ cup of water

¼ tsp of cinnamon

Preparation:

Combine the ingredients in a blender and pulse to combine.

Nutrition information per serving: Kcal: 98 Protein: 30g, Carbs: 26g, Fats: 4g, Sodium: 146mg

8.   Simply Vanilla Oats

Ingredients:

¾ cup of rolled oats

1 small apple, peeled and finely chopped

1 tsp of gluten-free vanilla extract

½ cup of almond milk

water

Preparation:

Place the oats in a bowl and cover with water. Allow it to stand for a while for the oats to soak well and soften. Drain and transfer to a pot.

Add chopped apple, mix with the oats, and pour about one cup of filtered water.

Bring to a boiling point and reduce the heat to minimum. Stir in the vanilla extract and almond milk. Mix well.

Cook for several minutes, stirring constantly.

When done, sprinkle with some cinnamon and serve.

Nutrition information per serving: Kcal: 226 Protein: 19g, Carbs: 21g, Fats: 7g, Sodium: 198mg

9.   Overnight Oaty Fun

Ingredients:
½ cup of gluten-free oats
1 cup of unsweetened almond milk
1 tsp of ground cinnamon
½ medium-sized apple, sliced
¼ cup of walnuts
1 tsp of maple syrup

Preparation:

Bring one cup of almond milk to a boiling point. Add the oats and briefly cook for several minutes. Reduce the heat to minimum and stir in ground cinnamon and maple syrup. Mix well and cook for several more minutes, or until the oats have soften.

Remove from the heat and cool for a while. Cover and leave in the refrigerator overnight.

Top with walnuts and sliced apple. You can drizzle some more maple syrup if necessary.

Nutrition information per serving: Kcal: 220 Protein: 14g, Carbs: 35g, Fats: 11g, Sodium: 230mg

10. Whipped Cream Parfait

Ingredients:

2 cups of strawberries

1 cup of whipped cream

¼ cup of walnuts

Preparation:

Wash the strawberries, clean and finely chop. Slightly beat the cream.

Take a few pieces of strawberries for decoration, and lightly mash the rest.

Make layers in the serving cup. First you need one layer of flakes. Continue with a layer of whipped cream and end with a layer of berries. Repeat the process until you have used all materialGarnish with chopped walnuts and strawberries.

Nutrition information per serving: Kcal: 90 Protein: 26g, Carbs: 29g, Fats: 5g, Sodium: 150mg

11. Sugar-Free Muffins

Ingredients:

1 cup of oat bran

1 cup of whole wheat or rye flour

1 tsp of baking powder

1 tsp of vanilla powder, sugar-free

2 tbsp of cold-pressed sunflower oil

2 tbsp of Stevia

3 tablespoons of water

1 egg

2 tbsp of lemon juice

1 cup of blueberries

Preparation:

Preheat oven to 350 °. Grease the muffin molds and set aside.

Mix oat bran, flour, baking powder and vanilla powder in a bowl.

Combine oil, Stevia, water, egg and lemon juice. Gently whisk in this mixture into the dry mixture. Stir in blueberries and lemon rind.

Pour into molds and bake for 15 minutes.

Nutrition information per serving: Kcal: 317 Protein: 21.5g, Carbs: 39g, Fats: 18g, Sodium: 361mg

12. Oatmeal with Blackberries and Agave Syrup

Ingredients:

1 cup of rolled oats

½ cup of blackberries

1 tsp of agave syrup

Preparation:

Place the oats in a bowl and cover with water. Allow it to stand for a while for the oats to soak well and soften. Drain and transfer to a pot. Add enough water to cover and bring it to a boil. Cook for five minutes.

Transfert to a serving bowl and stir in agave syrup and top with blackberries.

Nutrition information per serving: Kcal: 219 Protein: 8.7g, Carbs: 29g, Fats: 5.9g, Sodium: 187mg

13.   Scrambled Eggs with Raspberries

Ingredients:

2 eggs

½ cup of raspberries

1 tsp of agave syrup

2 tbsp of sugar-free whipped cream

2 tbsp of olive oil

Preparation:

Heat up the olive oil over medium-high heat.

Whisk the eggs and fry for 2 minutes, stirring constantly.

In a small bowl, combine taspberries with agave syrup and whipped cream. Use to top eggs or serve separately.

Nutrition information per serving: Kcal: 189 Protein: 34g, Carbs: 19g, Fats: 21g, Sodium: 206mg

14.   Avocado Eggs with Dry Rosemary

Ingredients:

3 medium ripe avocados, cut in half

6 eggs

1 medium tomato, finely chopped

3 tbsp of olive oil

2 tsp of dried rosemary

salt and pepper to taste

Preparation:

Preheat oven to 350 degrees. Cut avocado in half and remove the flesh from the center. Place one egg and chopped tomato in each avocado half and sprinkle with rosemary, salt and pepper. Grease the baking pan with olive oil and place the avocados. You want to use a small baking pan so your avocados can fit tightly. Place in the oven for about 15-20 minutes.

Nutrition information per serving: Kcal: 280 Protein: 28g, Carbs: 41g, Fats: 20g, Sodium: 303mg

15.   Creamy Lunch Pancakes To-Go

Ingredients:

1 cup of all purpose flour

2 eggs

½ tsp of salt

1 tbsp of sour cream

2 tsp of baking powder

1 cup of skim milk

1 cup of cottage cheese

1 cup of spinach, cooked and drained

non-fat cooking spray

Preparation:

Combine the flour, eggs, salt, sour cream, baking powder, and 1 cup of milk in a bowl. Mix well with an electric mixer until nice and smooth mixture. Cover it and let it stand for 15 minutes.

In another bowl, mix the cottage cheese with drained spinach. Beat well with a fork. Set aside.

Sprinkle some non-fat cooking spray on a frying pan. Use ¼ cup of dough mixture to make one thin pancake. Fry your pancakes for about 10-15 seconds on each side. This mixture should give you 6 pancakes.

Spread 1 tbsp of cheese mixture over each pancake and serve.

Nutrition information per serving: Kcal: 302 Protein: 36g, Carbs: 18g, Fats: 18g, Sodium: 355mg

16. Sweet Potatoes with Egg Whites

Ingredients:

4 medium sweet potatoes, peeled

6 eggs

2 medium onions, peeled

1 tbsp of ground garlic

4 tbsp of olive oil

½ tsp of sea salt

¼ tsp of ground pepper

Preparation:

Preheat your oven to 350 degrees. Spread 2 tbsp of olive oil over a medium sized baking sheet. Place the potatoes on a baking sheet. Bake for about 20 minutes. Remove from the oven and allow it to cool for a while. Lover the oven heat to 200 degrees.

Meanwhile, chop the onions into small pieces. Separate egg whites from yolks. Cut the potatoes into thick slices and place them in a bowl. Add chopped onions, 2 tbsp of olive oil, egg whites, ground garlic, sea salt and pepper. Mix well.

Spread this mixture over a baking sheet and bake for another 15-20 minutes.

Nutrition information per serving: Kcal: 390 Protein: 38g, Carbs: 40g, Fats: 26g, Sodium: 380mg

17. Spinach Ravioli

Ingredients:

<u>Ravioli</u>

2 ½ cups of all purpose flour

½ cups of water

3 eggs

3 egg whites

½ tsp of salt

3 tbsp of olive oil

<u>Filling</u>

2 tbsp of olive oil

2 cups of spinach, chopped

1 cup of cottage cheese

1 cup of low fat yogurt

¼ tsp of salt

¼ tsp of pepper

Preparation:

In a large bowl, combine all purpose flour, water, eggs, olive oil and salt. You want to make a smooth dough. Cover and let it stand in a warm place for about 30 minutes.

Briefly boil spinach in salted water, drain and cut. Combine with cottage cheese, yogurt, oil, salt and pepper.

Roll the dough thinly, cut out circles using molds and put in each hemisphere spoon of stuffing. Replace the second part of dough and press the edges with a fork so that the stuffing does not fall off.

Cook ravioli in boiling water to which you have added a little salt and olive oil. It should take about 15 minutes. Remove from the saucepan and drain. Serve with some low fat cream on top (this is optional).

Nutrition information per serving: Kcal: 390 Protein: 41g, Carbs: 45g, Fats: 26g, Sodium: 398mg

18.   Light Mac and Tuna

Ingredients:

1 cup of minced tuna

½ cup of low fat sour cream

2 cups of rice flour macaroni

1 tsp of sea salt

1 tsp of olive oil

1 tbsp of vegetable oil

Few olives for decoration (optional)

Preparation:

Pour 3 cups of water in a pot. Bring it to boil and add macaroni and salt. Boil macaroni for about 3 minutes (rice flour macaroni take less time to cook). You can also use the package instructions to cook macaroni, if you're not sure. Remove from heat and drain.

In a bowl, combine tuna with low fat sour cream. Mash well with a fork.

In a large saucepan, melt 1 tsp of olive oil and add 1 tbsp of vegetable oil. Heat up over a medium temperature and add tuna mixutre. Fry for about 15-20 minutes stirring occasionaly. Add macaroni and mix well. Cover the saucepan and allow maccaroni to heat up. Serve warm with some olives.

Nutrition information per serving: Kcal: 350 Protein: 36g, Carbs: 38g, Fats: 18g, Sodium: 340mg

19. Chicken Thighs

Ingredients:

2 pounds of chicken thighs

2 medium onions, chopped

2 small chili peppers

1 cup of chicken broth

¼ cup of freshly squeezed orange juice, unsweetened

1 tsp of orange extract, sugar-free

2 tbsp of olive oil

1 tsp of barbecue seasoning mix

1 small red onion, chopped

Preparation:

Heat up the olive oil in a large saucepan. Add chopped onions and fry for several minutes, over a medium temperature – until golden color.

Combine chili peppers, orange juice and orange extract. Mix well in a food processor for 20-30 seconds. Add this mixture into a saucepan and stir well. Reduce heat to simmer.

Coat the chicken with barbecue seasoning mix and put into a saucepan. Add chicken broth and bring it to boil. Cook over a medium temperature until the water evaporates. Remove from the heat.

Preheat the oven to 350 degrees. Place the chicken into a large baking dish. Bake for about 15 minutes to get a nice crispy, golden brown color.

Nutrition information per serving: Kcal: 180 Protein: 41g, Carbs: 14g, Fats: 30g, Sodium: 80mg

20. Grilled Veal Steak with Vegetables

Ingredients:

1 pound of veal steak, about 1 inch thick

1 medium red pepper

1 medium green pepper

1 small onion, finely chopped

3 tbsp of olive oil

Salt and pepper to taste

Preparation:

Wash and pat dry the steak with a kitchen paper. Heat up the olive oil over a medium temperature in a non-stick grill pan and fry for about 20 minutes (about 10 on each side). Remove from the heat and set aside.

Wash and cut vegetables into thin strips. Add some salt and pepper. Add to a grill pan and cook for about 15 minutes stirring constantly.

Serve immediately.

Nutrition information per serving: Kcal: 350 Protein: 39g, Carbs: 32g, Fats: 18g, Sodium: 111mg

21.   Chicken and Rice

Ingredients:

1 pound of chicken thighs

1 cup of brown rice

3 cups of chicken broth

1 small onion, chopped

1 large carrot, chopped

½ cup of artichoke, cooked

½ cup of green beans, cooked and drained

½ tsp of salt

¼ tsp of peper

Preparation:

Place the chicken in a deep pot. Add the onions and broth to cover about half of the meat. Bring it to a boil and cook over a medium heat until the meat is soft. Remove from the heat and transfer to a baking dish.

Add the remaining ingredients and mix well until thoroughly combined.

Preheat oven to 250 degrees. Bake covered for about 30 minutes, or until rice is done, stirring it several times during cooking.

Nutrition information per serving: Kcal: 209 Protein: 45g, Carbs: 42g, Fats: 24g, Sodium: 189mg

22.   Pan Roasted Lamb with Rice

Ingredients:

2 pounds of lamb cutlets, boneless

1 cup of rice

2 ½ cup of water

1 tsp of ground turmeric

5 tbsp of olive oil

¼ cup of freshly squeezed lemon juice

3 cloves of garlic, minced

½ tsp of sea salt

½ tsp of ground pepper

1 tbsp of all-purpose flour

¼ cup of water

Preparation:

Boil 2 ½ cup of water and add rice. Cook over medium temperature for about 10 minutes, or until the water evaporates. Remove from the heat and add ground turmeric. This will give your rice a nice golden color but it will also add some amazing nutritional values to your food. Cover the rice and set aside.

Wash and pat dry the cutlets. Heat up the olive oil over a medium temperature. Add the cutlets into a skillet and cook for about 10 minutes on each side. Reduce the heat to low and add flour, minced garlic, lemon juice, salt, pepper and some more water (¼ cup should be enough). Stir well and cook for about 15 minutes.

Serve with rice.

Nutrition information per serving: Kcal: 355 Protein: 46g, Carbs: 42g, Fats: 31g, Sodium: 389mg

23.   Crispy Salmon Slices

Ingredients:

1 pound of fresh salmon, sliced into 1 inch slices

1 cup of sour cream

1 cup of Greek yogurt

1 tbsp of garlic powder

2 eggs

½ tsp of sea salt

1 tbsp of dry parsley

2 tbsp of canola oil

Preparation:

Combine the sour cream, Greek yogurt, eggs, garlic powder, salt, and dry parsley in a bowl. Place almond slices in it, cover and marinate for about an hour.

Preheat the oven to 350 degrees. Pour the almond slices along with marinade in a small baking dish. Bake for 35 minutes. Remove from the oven, and serve with marinade.

Nutrition values per serving:

Nutrition information per serving: Kcal: 388 Protein: 39g, Carbs: 28g, Fats: 26g, Sodium: 180mg

SUGAR-FREE SNACKS

24.   Fresh Strawberry Pancakes

Ingredients:

1 cup of all purpose flour

2 eggs

2 tsp of sugar

1 tsp of vanilla extract, sugar-free

1 tbsp of sour cream

2 tsp of baking powder

1 cup of skim milk

1 cup of fresh strawberries

2 tbsp of oil for frying

Preparation:

Combine all dry ingredients in a large bowl. Mix well and gently whisk in 1 cup of milk, 2 eggs and 1 tbsp of sour cream. Cover and let it stand for about 7-10 minutes.

Meanwhile, pour some oil in a medium, nonstick frying pan and preheat over a medium temperature. About 1 tbsp of oil will be enough for the first two pancakes. You can add some more oil later. Pour some pancake mixture onto the frying pan. Fry for about a minute on one side, flip and fry for another minute on other side, or until light brown color on both sides. Transfer to a plate.

Top each pancake with fresh strawberries and serve.

Nutrition information per serving: Kcal: 300 Protein: 15g, Carbs: 40g, Fats: 16g, Sodium: 355mg

25.   Cheese Sticks

Ingredients:

1 cup of all-purpose flour

1/2 tbsp of baking powder

1 egg

1 tbsp of margarine

1 cup of grated Gouda cheese

½ cup of skim milk

Oil for frying

Preparation:

Combine in a bolw and use an electric mixer to make a smooth dough. Make a smooth dough. Roll out and cut into 1 inch thick sticks.

Preheat ½ cup of oil in a deep frying skillet, over high heat. Add cheese sticks and fry for a couple of minutes.

Use some kitchen paper to soak up the excess oil.

Serve warm.

Nutrition information per serving: Kcal: 412 Protein: 41g, Carbs: 35g, Fats: 26g, Sodium: 487mg

26.   Fruit Cupcakes

Ingredients:

Cupcake dough mix (refrigerated)

For the glaze:

1 cup of honey

½ cup of stevia

Sliced vegetables of your choice

Preparation:

Preheat the oven to 300 degrees F. Place the cupcake liner in a baking sheet. Add two tablespoons of cupcake dough onto the botton of each cupcake. Bake for about 20 minutes, at 300 degrees. Remove from the oven and arrange the fruits on top. Whisk together the glaze ingredients in a small bowl. Pour the mixture over the cupcakes and bake for another 5-6 minutes.

Nutrition information per serving: Kcal: 312 Protein: 36g, Carbs: 44g, Fats: 29g, Sodium: 690mg

27. Oat Cookies

Ingredients:

1 ½ cup of rolled oats plus

½ cup of peanut butter

¼ cup of minced almonds

3 tablespoons of agave syrup

1 tablespoon of minced chia seeds

1 tbsp of vanilla extract, sugar-free

3 cups of skim milk

Preparation:

Place one cup of rolled oats in a bowl. Add other dry ingredients and stir to combine.

Now add in peanut butter and agave syrup. Mix well and gently pour in the milk and vanilla extract. Shape the cookins using your hands, place in preheated oven. Bake at 350 degrees for 20 minutes.

Nutrition information per serving: Kcal: 320

Protein: 41g, Carbs: 56g, Fats: 19g, Sodium: 519mg

28.   Cheese Spread

Ingredients:

a cup of fresh cottage cheese

1 cup of cream

spices and herbs to taste (onions, chives, red pepper, fresh basil, etc)

a little salt and pepper

2 slices of whole wheat bread

Preparation:

Mix the cheese and sour cream, add the spices that the child likes and mix well. You can serve the dish or as a spread.

Nutrition information per serving: Kcal: 340 Protein: 44g, Carbs: 59g, Fats: 21g, Sodium: 615mg

29. Homemade Apple Puree

Ingredients:

5-6 medium sized apples (Alkmene apple)

1 tsp of ground cinnamon

6 tbsp of Stevia

4 cups of water

Preparation:

Wash and peel the apples. Cut into quarters and remove the core. Place them in a large pot and pour enough water to cover them (4 cups will do the job). Bring them to a boiling point and keep cooking until soft. Stir occasionally. After about 20 minutes, remove from the heat and drain. Allow it to cool for a while and mash with a fork. Add Stevia and ground cinnamon.

Refrigerate for 30 minutes before serving.

Nutrition information per serving: Kcal: 98 Protein: 7g, Carbs: 38g, Fats: 5g, Sodium: 140mg

30.   Fruit Balls

Ingredients:

1 cup of minced almonds

½ cup of peanut butter

½ cup of agave syrup

2 tablespoons of minced chia seeds

¼ cup of raw cocoa powder, unsweetened

¼ cup of grated dark chocolate, sugar-free

¼ cup of milk

Preparation:

Combine the ingredients in a bowl and mix well to combine. Shape the balls using your hands and refrigerate for about 30 minutes.

Nutrition information per serving: Kcal: 360 Protein: 11.5g, Carbs: 42g, Fats: 18g, Sodium: 414mg

31.   Creamy Yogurt Breakfast

Ingredients:

1 cup of Turkish yogurt

1 tbsp of low-fat whipped cream, unsweetened

1 egg white

2 tsp of honey

½ tsp of vanilla extract, sugar-free

Preparation:

For this easy recipe, combine 1 tbsp of whipped cream with 1 cup of Turkish yogurt, 1 egg white, ½ tsp of vanilla extract and 2 tbsp of honey. Use a fork or an electric mixer to get a smooth mixture. Allow it to cool in the refrigerator.

Nutrition information per serving: Kcal: 119 Protein: 33g, Carbs: 7g, Fats: 17g, Sodium: 150mg

32.   Fruit Salad

Ingredients

1 cup of fruits of your choice, sliced (We used apple, peach, grapes, blueberries and lime)

2 tbsp of low fat whipped cream

1 tbsp of honey

Preparation:

Combine the fruits in a large bowl. Add honey and mix well. Top with whipped cream. Serve cold.

Nutrition information per serving: Kcal: 190 Protein: 21g, Carbs: 44g, Fats: 12g, Sodium: 143mg

33.   Avocado Salsa

Ingredients:

2 ripe avocados, pitted and diced

½ cup of minced onions

2 jalapeno peppers, seeded and minced

3 organic limes, juiced

2 tbsp of extra virgin olive oil

2 tbsp of minced fresh cilantro leaves

Salt and crushed black pepper, to taste

Preparation:

Combine together all salsa ingredients in a large bowl and mix well with an electric mixer. Cover and chill until needed.

Nutrition information per serving: Kcal: 219 Protein: 17g, Carbs: 44g, Fats: 24g, Sodium: 180mg

34. Mashed Cauliflower

Ingredients:

2 cups of cauliflower, chopped

fresh water

½ cup of skim milk

1 tbsp of Greek yogurt, sugar-free

salt

1 tsp of dry mint (or any other seasoning of your choice)

Preparation:

Wash and roughly chop the cauliflower. Cook for about 15-20 minutes in salted water. When done, drain and mash it with a fork. Add milk, Greek yogurt, and mix well until smooth mixture. I always do this with an electric mixer. Add some more salt if you want and sprinkle with dry mint.

Nutrition information per serving: Kcal: 119 Protein: 36g, Carbs: 19g, Fats: 17g, Sodium: 121mg

35. Egg and Avocado Puree

Ingredients:

2 eggs

1 cup of low-fat milk

1 tbsp of sour cream

1 ripe avocado

few mint leaves

salt to taste

Preparation:

Hard boil your eggs. Remove from the heat and allow it to cool. Peel and cut the eggs. Add a pinch of salt and leave in the refrigerator for about 30 minutes. Meanwhile, peel and chop avocado. Place it in a blender. Add milk, eggs, cream and mint leaves. Mix well for about 30 seconds. Serve cold.

Nutrition information per serving: Kcal: 216 Protein: 35g, Carbs: 39g, Fats: 28g, Sodium: 189mg

36.   Kale Chips

Ingredients:

1 tablespoon Himalayan Crystal Salt

1 bunch of kale

Preparation:

Preheat your oven to 350 degrees. Take a baking sheet and line it with parchment paper. Use a knife to remove the leaves from the kale. Make sure you don't get any of the stem. Cut the leaves down into chewable, bite-size pieces. Wash the kale.

Bake the kale until the edges are brown and apply the salt to taste. This shouldn't take more than 15 minutes.

Nutrition information per serving: Kcal: 89 Protein: 2.9g, Carbs: 28g, Fats: 0.4g, Sodium: 140mg

37.   Fruit Pizza

Ingredients:

2 pears

1 apple

1 cup ofstrawberries

few slices ofpineapple

1 cup of peaches, cherries, figs (optional)

½ cup of skim milk

1 Pizza dough

1 orange

1 lemon

1 cup whipping cream, sugar-free

Preparation:

Use package instructions to prepare the dough.

Wash and clean the fruits. Peel the pineapple and figs and cut them into cubes, then cut orange and lemon with rind.

Mix the whipping cream with milk until smooth. Roll out the dough and divide it into four rounds that will smear the mixture of milk and cream.

Bake for 15 minutes at 350°.

Remove the pizza from the oven and decorate them with prepared fruit. Return to the oven for another five minutes.

Nutrition information per serving: Kcal: 440 Protein: 25g, Carbs: 51g, Fats: 21g, Sodium: 419mg

38.   Mixed Wild Berries Salad

Ingredients:

1 cup of mixed wild berries

1 banana

1 apple

Preparation:

Cut and peel the apple and banana. Cut them into small pieces and mix with berries. Cool well before serving.

Nutrition information per serving: Kcal: 225 Protein: 3g, Carbs: 35g, Fats: 0.9g, Sodium: 162mg

39. Vegetables in Honey Wok

Ingredients:

1 pound of chicken breast, boneless and skinless

1 medium red pepper, cut into strips

1 medum green pepper, cut into strips

7-8 pieces of baby corn

½ cup of canned button mushrooms

1 cup of cauliflower

1 medium carrot, peeled and cut into strips

1 tsp honey

Salt to taste

1 tbsp of olive oil

Preparation:

Cut the meat into bite size pieces.

In a large wok, heat up the olive oil over a high temperature. Add the chicken meat and cook for about 10 minutes stirring constantly. Remove from the wok. Now you have to cook the vegetables. First add carrot strips and cauliflower. They take the most time to soften. Now add red and green pepper strips, baby corn, button mushrooms, and honey. Cook for another 5-7 minutes. You don't want to overcook the vegetables. It has to stay crispy. Add the meat, mix well and serve with rice.

Nutrition information per serving: Kcal: 319 Protein: 45g, Carbs: 47g, Fats: 29g, Sodium: 468mg

40.   Mushroom Steak

Ingredients:

1 ½ pounds of beef flank steaks

2 tbsp of vegetable oil

½ tsp of salt

2 cups of button mushrooms

Preparation:

Wash and pat dry the steaks with kitchen paper.

In a large skillet, heat up the vegetable oil over a medium temperature. Fry the steaks for about 5-7 minutes on each side. Reduce the heat to low and add mushrooms. Cover the skillet and cook for another few minutes. Serve warm.

Nutrition information per serving: Kcal: 345 Protein: 51g, Carbs: 12g, Fats: 28g, Sodium: 169mg

41.   Heavy Winter Stew

Ingredients:

2 pounds of stew beef

1 tablespoon of vegetable oil

6 ounces tomato paste

2 carrots, cut into strips

1 large tomato, chopped

1 large onion, chopped

1 cup of button mushrooms

¼ tbsp of salt

1 bay leaf

2 ½ cups beef broth

1 tsp of dry thyme

3 minced garlic cloves

Preparation:

Take a frying pan and set it over high heat. Heat up the vegetable oil and add the beef to it. Fry the beef on both sides until properly brown. Once the beef is lightly brown, transfer it to the slow cooker. In the same pan, fry the onions, turning the heat to medium. Cook the onions for around 5 minutes.

Pour the tomato paste in the frying pan to scoop up any remaining bits of the beef and onions. After this, pour the mixture over the beef in a deep pot. Put in all the remaining ingredients and stir properly, especially if the liquid is thick. Cover the pot, set the heat to low and cook for about an hour.

Nutrition information per serving: Kcal: 416 Protein: 51g, Carbs: 42g, Fats: 32g, Sodium: 557mg

42. Cheesy Muffins

Ingredients:

2 cups of all purpose flour

1 tbsp of baking powder

½ tsp of salt

1 cup of milk

2 eggs

¼ cup of olive oil

¼ cup of cottage cheese

¼ cup of spinach, cooked and squeezeed

muffin molds

Preparation:

In a large bowl, combine all dry ingredients. Gently whisk in milk and crack 2 eggs. Mix well with an electric mixer. This will give you a nice, smooth muffin dough. Now add spinach and cheese into the dough and mix well again. Shape the muffins using muffin molds.

Preheat the oven to 300 degrees. Bake for about 25 minutes.

Nutrition information per serving: Kcal: 215 Protein: 27g, Carbs: 35g, Fats: 19g, Sodium: 199mg

43. Homemade Mayo Stuffed eggs

Ingredients:

6 eggs (large, hard-boiled, peeled)

2/3 cup of mayonnaise, homemade

2 tablespoons of dill pickles, chopped finely

¼ cup of celery, diced finely

¼ cup of onion, diced finely

1 cup of crab meat, cooked, picked out

1 tablespoon of vegetable seasoning

salt to taste

pepper to taste

Homemade mayonnaise

1 egg yolk (large)

¼ teaspoon of salt

¼ teaspoon of mustard

1 ½ tablespoon of freshly squeezed lemon juice

1 teaspoon of white vinegar

¾ cup of avocado oil (can use macadamia nut oil as well)

Preparation:

Homemade mayonnaise:

Take a large bowl and whisk the egg yolk, salt, mustard, lemon juice and white vinegar together until the egg yolk starts to change color and thicken. Slowly pour ¼ cup of the oil in the mixture as you whisk vigorously for 1 minute. Slowly pour ¼ cup more after 30 seconds of whisking and add the remaining oil at once and whisk everything, energetically, together until you get a thick, creamy, emulsified mayonnaise.

Stuffed eggs:

Cut the hard boiled eggs in half, lengthwise and use a small teaspoon to scoop out the cooked yolks carefully without damaging the whites. Set the whites aside and place all the yolks in a bowl. Add the pickle, celery, mayonnaise, onions, and some salt and pepper to the yolks in the bowls. Using the fork, mash the yolks and mix everything together until they are well combined.

Now, add the crab meat to the mixture and fold it in gently. Check seasoning and add more if needed. Pick up an egg white and add one spoonful of the mixture in the hollow area where you scooped out the yolk from and set aside on a tray. Fill all the yolks in this manner.

Nutrition information per serving: Kcal: 180 Protein: 48g, Carbs: 17g, Fats: 23g, Sodium: 214mg

44. Tomato Tostadas

Ingredients:

1 cup of cherry tomatoes, cut in half

1 cup of red cabbage, finely chopped

2 pieces of chicken breast, shredded into large pieces

½ cup of green beans, cooked

½ cup of corn, cooked

1 tbsp of chili sauce, sugar-free

½ tsp of salt

1 tsp of ground garlic

1 tsp of dry parsley

¼ tsp of ground black pepper

2 tbsp of fresh lemon juice

1 tbsp of stevia

1 tsp of dry oregano

3 tbsp of olive oil

4 tortillas

Preparation:

In a large skillet, combine the tomatoes, oregano and salt. Stir well and fry for 2-3 minutes, over a medium temperature. Season with pepper. Now you can add the meat and cook for about 10-15 minutes, until nice golden color. Add the remaining ingredients and cover. Let it stand for about 10 minutes.

Top each tortilla with chicken and vegetable mixture . Serve warm.

Nutrition information per serving: Kcal: 389 Protein: 31g, Carbs: 49g, Fats: 21g, Sodium: 414mg

45. Spinach Pie

Ingredients:

1 pack (9 ounces) of fresh spinach, chopped

4 whole eggs

½ cup of whole milk

2 ounces of crumbled Feta cheese

¼ cup grated Parmesan cheese

½ cup shredded Mozzarella cheese

1 teaspoon of olive oil

salt and black pepper, to taste

1 pack of pie crust

Preparation:

Preheat an oven to a temperature of 350°F. Lightly grease a baking dish with olive oil and set aside.

Place one pie crust on the bottom of your baking dish.

Whisk the eggs thoroughly in a mixing bowl, mix in the milk and grated Parmesan and whisk until well incorporated. Set aside.

Place the chopped spinach on the greased pie crust and add crumbled Feta cheese. Pour in the egg mixture and cover the other ingredients completely. Place another pie crust on top and bake for about 40 to 45 minutes or until the cheese has melted and lightly browned.

Remove from the oven and let it rest for 5 minutes before serving.

Nutrition information per serving: Kcal: 399 Protein: 42g, Carbs: 44g, Fats: 26g, Sodium: 415mg

46.   Lemon Shrimps

Ingredients:

1 pound of fresh shrimps

1 organic lemon, sliced into wedges for serving

1 tbsp of fresh rosemary, for serving

For the Marinade

4 tbsp extra virgin olive oil

1 tsp of minced garlic

2 tbsp of organic lemon juice

½ tsp of salt

½ tsp of crushed black pepper

½ tsp of dried thyme leaves

½ tsp of dried oregano

Preparation:

Combine together all marinade ingredients in a medium bowl and mix until well combined. Place the shrimp and coat evenly with the marinade mixture. Cover the bowl and chill for at least 1 hour to marinate the shrimps.

Preheat gas grill to high heat and brush the grids with oil. Insert 2 to 3 shrimps on each skewer, brush with marinade and grill for 3 minutes on each side. Turn to cook the other side for another 3 minutes and transfer into a serving platter.

Serve warm with lemons wedges and sprinkle with minced parsley.

Nutrition information per serving: Kcal: 219 Protein: 35g, Carbs: 19g, Fats: 19g, Sodium: 161mg

47.   Green Pizza

Ingredients:

1 medium whole wheat pizza crust

¼ cup of sugar free pizza sauce

½ cup of chopped spinach

1 small cucumber, cut into strips

½ small onion, chopped

1 cup of cottage cheese

¼ cup of gouda, grated

2 tbsp of grated parmesan cheese

1 tbsp of olive oil

Preparation:

Preheat the oven to 350 degrees. Lay the pizza crust on a baking sheet. Spread the sauce over the pizza crust. Now add the spinach and the onions. Sprinkle with cottage cheese and grated gouda. Make a final layer with parmesan. Drizzle the olive oil. Bake for about 10 mintes, cut and spread some cucmber strips on top. Serve immediately.

Nutrition information per serving: Kcal: 419 Protein: 28g, Carbs: 46g, Fats: 25g, Sodium: 660mg

48.   Grilled Tuna Steaks

Ingredients:

¼ cup of chopped fresh coriander leaves

3 garlic cloves, minced

2 tablespoons of lemon juice

½ cup olive oil

4 tuna steaks

½ teaspoon smoked paprika

½ teaspoon cumin, ground

½ teaspoon chili powder

Salt and black pepper

Preparation:

Add the coriander, garlic, paprika, cumin, chilli powder and lemon juice in a food processor and pulse to combine. Gradually add in the oil and mix the ingredients until a smooth mixture.

Transfer the mixture into a bowl, add the fish and gently toss to coat the fish evenly with sauce. Chill for at least 2 hours to allow the flavors to penetrate into the fish.

Remove the fish from the chiller and preheat the grill. Lightly brush the grid with oil, place the fish and grill for about 3 to 4 minutes on each side.

Remove the fish from the grill, transfer on a serving plate and serve with lemon wedges or some vegetables

Nutrition information per serving: Kcal: 350 Protein: 41g, Carbs: 12g, Fats: 19g, Sodium: 150mg

49.   Sugar-Free Coconut Dessert

Ingredients

1 can organic coconut milk

1 cup of mixed frozen berries

¼ cup of rolled oats

½ banana, peeled and sliced

2 tbsp of almonds, ground

1 tbsp of agave syrup

water

Preparation:

Combine the ingredients in a blender and pulse to combine for 30 seconds, or until smooth mixture.

Serve immediately.

You can add any some other fruits and create a combination your kid will love.

Nutrition information per serving: Kcal: 112 Protein: 23g, Carbs: 27g, Fats: 16g, Sodium: 156mg

50. Homemade Chocolate Chip Cookies

Ingredients:

1 cup of all-purpose flour

1 teaspoon of baking powder

1 cup of sugar substitute blend

A pinch of salt

2 tbsp of grated lemon zest

2 tbsp of olive oil

2 egg yolks

1 tbsp of lemon juice

2oz unsweetened dark chocolate (85% cocoa), finely chopped

Preparation:

Combine all dry ingredients in a medium-sized bowl. Gently whisk in the milk and add chocolate. Mix well until smooth dough. Refrigerate for 30 minutes.

Preheat the oven to 350 degrees. Place some baking paper over a baking sheet.

Roll out chilled dough on a floured surface until 2 inches thick. Using molds, shape the biscuits and transfer to a baking sheet. Cook for 20 minutes, or until browned.

Nutrition information per serving: Kcal: 212 Protein: 24g, Carbs: 46g, Fats: 18g, Sodium: 373mg

51.   Sugar-Free Donuts

Ingredients

1.5 cup of buckwheat flour

½ cup of rice flour

½ cup of powdered oats

1 tsp of baking powder

2 cups of unsweetened almond milk

2 eggs

¼ cup of Stevia

½ tsp of ground cinnamon

2 tbsp of olive oil

For the glaze:

½ cup of powdered Stevia

2 tbsp of powdered cocoa, sugar free

1 tsp of vanilla extract, sugar-free

¼ cup of almond milk

1 tbsp of olive oil

Prepration:

Combine buckwheat flour, rice flour, powdered oats, baking powder, stevia and cinnamon in a large bowl. Break two eggs into the bowl, add 2 cups of milk and olive oil. Mix well using an electric mixer. Cover and set aside for 10-15 minutes. Sprinkle some rice flour on work surface. Roll out the dough and shape your donuts. If the mixture is too sticky, gently sprinkle with some more rice flour.

Pour some oil in a deep saucepan (2-3 inches from the bottom) and heat up over a high temperature.

Meanwhile, prepare the glaze. Stir together the glaze ingredients in a small saucepan. Bring it to a boiling point and remove from the heat. Cover and set aside.

Fry donuts for about two minutes on each side, over a high temperature. Remove from the saucepan and soak the excess oil using a kitchen paper.

Dip each donut in a chocolate glaze and transfer to a plate. Serve warm or cold.

Nutrition information per serving: Kcal: 350 Protein: 31g, Carbs: 46g, Fats: 29g, Sodium: 490mg

52.   Fruit Cup

Ingredients:

½ cup of cottage cheese

½ cup of whipping cream

4oz mixed fruits of your choice (works fine with practically anything you have in your fridge)

1 tsp of vanilla extract, sugar-free

1 tsp of powdered Stevia

1 tbsp of non-fat dessert cream, sugar-free

Preparation:

In a small bowl, combine cottage cheese with whipping cream, dessert cream and vanilla extract. Stir in stevia and use an electric mixer to beat on medium speed until well combined.

Use to top the fruits.

Nutrition information per serving: Kcal: 209 Protein: 29g, Carbs: 35g, Fats: 7g, Sodium: 298mg

53.   Sugar-Free Cocoa Drink

Ingredients:

1 cup of coconut milk

1 tsp of raw cocoa, unsweetened

1 tsp of agave syrup

1 cup of sugar-free whipping cream

Preparation:

Combine the ingredients in a blender and mix well for 30 seconds.

Transfer to a microvawe and heat up for one minute on high heat.

Nutrition information per serving: Kcal: 88 Protein: 8.9g, Carbs: 10.5g, Fats: 3g, Sodium: 95mg

JUICES

1.   Blueberry Juice

Ingredients:

1 cup of fresh blueberries

1 small apple

2 carrots

1 head romaine lettuce

Preparation:

Run all ingredients through a juicer. Serve cold

Nutritional information per serving: Kcal: 228, Protein: 6.14g, Carbs: 66.8g, Fats: 1.95g

2.   Pear Juice

Ingredients:

1 medium-sized pear, roughly chopped

½ cup of fresh grapes

3 large oranges

1 cup of spinach, torn

A handful of ginger, finely chopped

Preparation:

Wash and thoroughly rinse the spinach. Set aside.

Peel and section the oranges.

Run all ingredients through a juicer. Serve cold

Nutritional information per serving: Kcal: 347, Protein: 6.52g, Carbs: 108.8g, Fats: 1.27g

3.   Green Detox Juice

Ingredients:

1 cup of chopped broccoli

A bunch of fresh spinach

½ cup of coconut water, unsweetened

2 lemons

1 medium-sized orange

1 tbsp of honey, raw

few mint leaves

Preparation:

Place chopped broccoli, fresh spinach, two lemons, and orange in a juicer. Squeeze the juice and combine with unsweetened coconut water.

Add one tablespoon of raw honey and mix well.

Decorate with a couple of mint leaves and serve cold.

Nutritional information per serving: Kcal: 171, Protein: 14.8g, Carbs: 54.5g, Fats: 2.17g

4.   Berry Blast Juice

Ingredients:

1 cup of blackberries

1 cup of blueberries

1 cup of raspberries

1 cup of strawberries

¼ cup of baby spinach

½ tsp of ground ginger

Preparation:

Run the ingredients through a juicer. Sprinkle with ground ginger and serve cold.

Nutritional information per serving: Kcal: 158, Protein: 5.9g, Carbs: 56.4g, Fats: 2.3g

5.   Melon and Strawberry Juice

Ingredients:

2 cups of fresh strawberries

14 oz melon, roughly chopped

2 cups of spinach, chopped

1 medium-sized banana

½ tsp of cinnamon

1 tsp of honey, raw

Preparation:

Run strawberries, spinach, melon, and banana through a juicer.

Whisk in one teaspoon of raw honey and season with cinnamon.

Serve cold.

Nutritional information per serving: Kcal: 349, Protein: 7.6g, Carbs: 104.9g, Fats: 3.2g

6.   Strawberries smoothie

Ingredients:

2 cups of strawberries, fresh

1 cup of blueberries, fresh

½ cup of coconut water, unsweetened

½ large blood orange

1 tsp of pure coconut sugar

Preparation:

Add ingredients in a juicer, combine with coconut water and whisk in one teaspoon of pure coconut sugar.

Serve cold.

Nutritional information per serving: Kcal: 246, Protein: 4.7g, Carbs: 74.2g, Fats: 1.7g

7.   Vanilla Raspberry Juice

Ingredients:

3 cups of raspberries, fresh

½ cup of coconut water, unsweetened

½ tsp of pure vanilla extract, sugar-free

Preparation:

Place raspberries in a juicer and squeeze. Transfer to a serving glass. Add coconut water and vanilla extract.

Serve cold.

Nutritional information per serving: Kcal: 136, Protein: 4.4g, Carbs: 51.7g, Fats: 2.4g

8.   Goji Juice

Ingredients:

10 oz broccoli, pre-cooked

1 cup of goji berries

1 large orange, peeled

1 large cucumber, peeled

1 tbsp of honey, raw

Preparation:

Run the ingredients through a juicer.

Whisk in honey and serve cold

Nutritional information per serving: Kcal: 193, Protein: 9.4g, Carbs: 66g, Fats: 1.7g

9.   Orange Mocha Juice

Ingredients:

½ cup of unsweetened chilled coffee

4 large oranges

1 tsp of pure vanilla extract, sugar-free

1 tsp of pure coconut sugar

Preparation:

Run oranges through a juicer.

Combine with chilled coffee and whisk in coconut sugar.

Add vanilla extract and serve cold.

Nutritional information per serving: Kcal: 292, Protein: 6.9g, Carbs: 96g, Fats: 2g

10.   Morning Carrot Juice

Ingredients:

3 large carrots

2 Alkamene apples

½ tsp of cinnamon, freshly ground

1 tbsp of honey, raw

Preparation:

Place carrots and apples in a juicer, one at the time. Squeeze the juice and transfer to a serving glass.

Add one tablespoon of honey and some cinnamon to taste.

Serve cold.

Nutritional information per serving: Kcal: 324, Protein: 3.4g, Carbs: 93g, Fats: 1.5g

11. Granny Smith Juice

Ingredients:

2 large Granny Smith apples, sliced and seeds removed

1 large grapefruit, peeled

1 tsp of honey, raw

½ tsp of ginger, freshly ground

Preparation:

Run the fruits through a juicer.

Add one teaspoon of honey and freshly ground ginger.

Serve cold.

Nutritional information per serving: Kcal: 299, Protein: 3.7g, Carbs: 88g, Fats: 1.1g

12.   Fresh Pineapple Juice

Ingredients:

1 cup of pineapple chunks

1 small apple, peeled and seeds removed

1 tsp of fresh mint leaves, finely chopped

¼ tsp of nutmeg, ground

Preparation:

Place the fruit in a juicer and squeeze.

Add ground nutmeg and mix well. Decorate with a couple of mint leaves and serve cold.

Nutritional information per serving: Kcal: 141, Protein: 1.5g, Carbs: 41.2g, Fats: 0.4g

13.   Blueberry and Banana Juice

Ingredients:

1 cup of blueberries

1 cup of blackberries

1 large banana, peeled

1 tsp of honey

½ tsp of cinnamon

Preparation:

Run the ingredients through a juicer.

Add one teaspoon of honey and cinnamon. Mix well and serve warm.

Nutritional information per serving: Kcal: 229, Protein: 4.5g, Carbs: 76.3g, Fats: 1.6g

14.   Thick Banana Juice

Ingredients:

2 large bananas

1 cup of grapes

1 tsp of pure vanilla extract, sugar-free

½ cup of coconut milk, sugar-free

Preparation:

Place bananas and grapes in a juicer. Juice and transfer to a serving glass.

Combine with coconut milk and pure vanilla extract. Serve cold.

Nutritional information per serving: Kcal: 293, Protein: 7.5g, Carbs: 77.9g, Fats: 4g

15.   Peppermint Juice

Ingredients:

3 large cucumbers, peeled

1 grapefruit, peeled

1 tsp of peppermint extract

1 tbsp of coconut sugar

Preparation:

Prepare the fruits and place in a juicer. Squeeze and add peppermint extract and coconut sugar.

Serve with some ice.

Nutritional information per serving: Kcal: 204, Protein: 7.7g, Carbs: 59g, Fats: 1.3g

16.   Flaxseed and Goji Juice

Ingredients:

1 large banana

1 cup of goji berries

1 tsp of flaxseed oil

A bunch of celery leaves

1 tbsp of honey, raw

Preparation:

Run the ingredients through a juicer. Whisk in one teaspoon of flaxseed oil and honey.

Serve with ice.

Nutritional information per serving: Kcal: 177, Protein: 6.5g, Carbs: 44.6g, Fats: 2.6g

17.   Pumpkin Juice

Ingredients:

1 cup of avocado chunks

10 oz sweet pumpkin chunks

½ tsp of cinnamon, freshly ground

¼ cup of water

Preparation:

Place the fruit in a juicer and squeeze.

Combine with some water and add cinnamon.

Stir well and serve cold.

Nutritional information per serving: Kcal: 256, Protein: 5.3g, Carbs: 27.8g, Fats: 22.3g

18.   Almond Honey Juice

Ingredients:

½ cup of almond milk, sugar-free

1 tbsp of honey, raw

1 large banana, peeled

3 large red oranges, peeled

1 tbsp of fresh mint leaves, finely chopped

Preparation:

Run oranges and banana through a juicer. Combine with sugar-free almond milk and add one tablespoon of honey.

Decorate with a couple of mint leaves and serve cold.

Nutritional information per serving: Kcal: 411, Protein: 11g, Carbs: 95g, Fats: 3.1g

19. Fresh Tomato Juice

Ingredients:

5 large tomatoes, peeled

1 cup of fresh raspberries

½ tsp of pure cherry extract, sugar-free

A couple of mint leaves

Preparation:

Run the ingredients through a juicer.

Add cherry extract and some mint to taste.

Serve immediately.

Nutritional information per serving: Kcal: 152, Protein: 9.4g, Carbs: 50g, Fats: 2.6g

20. Greek Pomegranate Juice

Ingredients:

1 cup of pomegranate seeds

1 cup of fresh blackberries

1 large cucumber

A handful of fresh parsley

Preparation:

Place the ingredients in a juicer and squeeze.

Serve cold.

Nutritional information per serving: Kcal: 143, Protein: 7.9g, Carbs: 44.8g, Fats: 2.5g

21.   Ginger and Kale Juice

Ingredients:

1 cup of kale, torn

1 cup of strawberries, fresh

½ tsp of ginger, ground

1 lemon, peeled

Preparation:

Run the ingredients through a juicer and serve cold.

Nutritional information per serving: Kcal: 120, Protein: 5.9g, Carbs: 38.6g, Fats: 1.8g

22.   Guava Juice

Ingredients:

1 whole guava

1 cup of parsnip

1 celery stalk

2 large grapefruits, peeled

Preparation:

Juice and serve cold.

Nutritional information per serving: Kcal: 279, Protein: 7.2g, Carbs: 86g, Fats: 1.7g

23.   Butternut Squash Juice

Ingredients:

1 medium-sized banana, peeled

1 cup of raspberries, fresh

1 cup of butternut squash cubes

½ cup of coconut water, unsweetened

1 tsp of honey, raw

Preparation:

Run the ingredients through a juicer and combine with coconut water.

Whisk in one teaspoon of honey and serve cold.

Nutritional information per serving: Kcal: 197, Protein: 4.7g, Carbs: 68g, Fats: 1.3g

24.   Green Kiwi Juice

Ingredients:

3 large kiwis, peeled

1 cup of kale, torn

1 cup of cranberries

1 tsp of pure coconut sugar

Preparation:

Place kiwi, kale, and cranberries in a juicer. Squeeze and transfer to a serving glass.

Add one teaspoon of coconut sugar and serve cold.

Nutritional information per serving: Kcal: 153, Protein: 5.6g, Carbs: 48.4g, Fats: 1.8g

25.   Summer Coconut Juice

Ingredients:

½ cup of coconut water

1 cup of pineapple chunks

1 cup of mango chunks

1 cup of guava chunks

1 tbsp of fresh mint leaves

Preparation:

Juice and sprinkle with fresh mint.

Serve cold.

Nutritional information per serving: Kcal: 187, Protein: 3.6g, Carbs: 54.2g, Fats: 1.3g

26.   Mango Lime Juice

Ingredients:

1 cup of mango chunks

1 whole lime

1 cup of chard, torn

1 cup of beet greens, torn

½ cup of coconut water, unsweetened

Preparation:

Place the ingredients in a juicer and squeeze.

Combine with unsweetened coconut water and serve cold.

Nutritional information per serving: Kcal: 108, Protein: 3.8g, Carbs: 33g, Fats: 0.8g

27.   Energy Juice

Ingredients:

2 large Red Delicious apples, peeled and seeds removed

1 cup of goji berries

1 cup of fresh cherries, pitted

1 cup of beets

3 large tomatoes, peeled

Preparation:

Run the ingredients through a juicer and serve immediately.

Nutritional information per serving: Kcal: 328, Protein: 9.3g, Carbs: 95g, Fats: 2.14g

28. Fresh Aronia Juice

Ingredients:

2 cups of fresh aronia

1 large banana, peeled

2 cups of spinach, torn

2 cups of beet greens, torn

Preparation:

Place the ingredients in a juicer, one at the time.

Squeeze and serve immediately.

Nutritional information per serving: Kcal: 183, Protein: 7.8g, Carbs: 63.1g, Fats: 1.2g

29.   Green Apple and Carrot Juice

Ingredients:

2 large green apples, peeled and seeds removed

3 large carrots

1 cup of parsnip slices

1 basil leaf, crushed

¼ cup of water

Preparation:

Place the ingredients in a juicer and squeeze.

Combine with water and crushed basil.

Serve cold.

Nutritional information per serving: Kcal: 332, Protein: 5.4g, Carbs: 100g, Fats: 1.6g

30.   Avocado Juice

Ingredients:

1 whole avocado, chopped

7 oz artichoke

1 medium-sized lemon, peeled

1 cup of red cabbage, shredded

1 cup of green cabbage, shredded

Preparation:

Run the ingredients through a juicer and serve immediately.

Nutritional information per serving: Kcal: 353, Protein: 12.3g, Carbs: 51g, Fats: 30g

31.   Pineapple and Apricot Juice

Ingredients:

1 cup of pineapple chunks

1 cup of apricots

1 large cucumber, sliced

1 cup of fresh spinach, torn

1 whole lemon

½ cup of raw broccoli, chopped

½ cup of pure coconut water

Preparation:

Wash and prepare the ingredients.

Run through a juicer and combine with pure coconut water.

Serve immediately with ice.

Nutritional information per serving: Kcal: 218, Protein: 10g, Carbs: 64g, Fats: 1.9g

32.   Peachy Asparagus Juice

Ingredients:

1 large peach

1 cup of fresh asparagus, chopped

1 cup of collard greens

1 large grapefruit, peeled

1 cup of romaine lettuce, shredded

1 cup of fennel, sliced

Preparation:

Wash and slice the ingredients. Place in a juicer and squeeze.

Serve immediately.

Nutritional information per serving: Kcal: 187, Protein: 9.1g, Carbs: 57.9g, Fats: 1.4g

33.   Plum Power Juice

Ingredients:

1 cup of plums, halved

1 cup of fresh blackberries

1 cup of turnip greens, chopped

½ tsp of ground ginger

1 tsp of coconut sugar

½ cup of water

Preparation:

Wash and slice each plum in half. Run through a juicer.

Now juice blackberries and turnip greens.

Combine in a tall serving glass. Add ground ginger and coconut sugar.

Mix well and serve.

Nutritional information per serving: Kcal: 141, Protein: 4.2g, Carbs: 40.3g, Fats: 1.4g

34.   Lemon Juice

Ingredients:

3 large lemons, peeled

1 large orange, peeled

10 oz radish

1 cup of beet greens, chopped

1 cup of watercress, chopped

1 tbsp of honey, raw

Preparation:

Peel the fruits and run through a juicer. Add radish, beet greens, and watercress. Juice and add one tablespoon of honey.

Serve cold.

Nutritional information per serving: Kcal: 147, Protein: 5.3g, Carbs: 50g, Fats: 0.8g

35.   Cherry Mint Juice

Ingredients:

2 cups of cherries, pitted

1 cup of leek, chopped

1 tbsp of fresh mint, finely chopped

1 cup of fresh cranberries

1 tbsp of honey, raw

Preparation:

Run the ingredients through a juicer.

Add one tablespoon of honey and mix well.

Serve immediately.

Nutritional information per serving: Kcal: 248, Protein: 5g, Carbs: 75.5g, Fats: 1g

36.   Leafy Ginger Juice

Ingredients:

1 cup of beet greens, chopped

1 cup of cauliflower, chopped

1 cup of fennel, sliced

1 cup of celery, chopped

1 cup of red leaf lettuce, shredded

1 cup of romaine lettuce, shredded

1 large grapefruit

½ cup of pure coconut water

1 tsp of honey

Preparation:

Wash and prepare the ingredients. Run through a juicer and add one teaspoon of honey.

Serve cold.

Nutritional information per serving: Kcal: 163, Protein: 8.3g, Carbs: 56.3g, Fats: 1.2g

37.   Sweet Mango Juice

Ingredients:

1 cup of mango, chopped

1 cup of apricots, sliced

½ cup of pure coconut water, unsweetened

1 tbsp of coconut sugar

Preparation:

Wash and slice the fruits. Juice and combine with unsweetened coconut water.

Add one tablespoon of coconut sugar.

Serve cold.

Nutritional information per serving: Kcal: 155, Protein: 3.6g, Carbs: 43g, Fats: 1.2g

38.   Apple and Peach Juice

Ingredients:

2 large golden delicious apples, peeled and seeds removed

1 large peach, chopped

1 cup of baby spinach, torn

½ cup of water

1 large carrot

½ lemon

Preparation:

Run through a juicer and serve immediately.

Nutritional information per serving: Kcal: 297, Protein: 5.5g, Carbs: 87.5g, Fats: 1.5g

39.   Fresh Ginger Juice

Ingredients:

1 large banana, peeled

1 cup of spinach, torn

2 large lemons, peeled

1 slice of ginger

1 tsp of honey

Preparation:

Place the ingredients in a juicer, one at the time.

Juice and add honey.

Serve immediately.

Nutritional information per serving: Kcal: 139, Protein: 4.5g, Carbs: 44.4g, Fats: 1.2g

40.   Papaya Juice

Ingredients:

1 cup of papaya, chopped

1 cup of goji berries

1 cup of purple cabbage, shredded

1 large blood orange, peeled

1 tsp of ginger, ground

1 tsp of honey

Preparation:

Wash and chop the ingredients. Place in a juicer, one at the time and squeeze.

Add one teaspoon of ginger and one teaspoon of honey before serving.

Nutritional information per serving: Kcal: 172, Protein: 4.3g, Carbs: 54.2g, Fats: 0.7g

41.   Blueberry Juice

Ingredients:

1 cup of blueberries

2 large alkamene apples, cored and sliced

¼ cup of blackberries

1 tsp of pure mint extract, sugar-free

½ cup of water

Preparation:

Run through a juicer and serve immediately.

Nutritional information per serving: Kcal: 368, Protein: 2.5g, Carbs: 94g, Fats: 1.5g

42.   Pumpkin and Banana Juice

Ingredients:

1 cup of pumpkin cubes

1 large banana, peeled

1 large granny smith apple, peeled and cored

½ cup of pure coconut water, unsweetened

¼ tsp of nutmeg, ground

1 tbsp of coconut sugar

Preparation:

Peel and chop pumpkin. Run through a juicer.

Now add banana and apple, one at the time.

Combine with pure coconut water in a serving glass.

Add nutmeg and coconut sugar.

Serve immediately.

Nutritional information per serving: Kcal: 338, Protein: 4.6g, Carbs: 97.8g, Fats: 1.4g

43.   Raspberry Lime Juice

Ingredients:

1 cup of fresh raspberries

2 limes, peeled

2 cups of raw broccoli, chopped

½ cup of coconut water, unsweetened

2 large cucumbers, peeled

1 tbsp of honey, raw

Preparation:

Run the ingredients through a juicer.

Add one tablespoon of honey and mix well.

Serve immediately.

Nutritional information per serving: Kcal: 192, Protein: 10.9g, Carbs: 56g, Fats: 2.2g

44.   Honeydew Melon Juice

Ingredients:

1 large wedge of honeydew melon

1 large radish

1 cup of chard

1 cup of asparagus

1 cup of avocado, sliced

¼ cup of pure coconut water, unsweetened

Preparation:

Wash and prepare the ingredients.

Run through a juicer and combine with unsweetened coconut water.

Serve immediately.

Nutritional information per serving: Kcal: 275, Protein: 8g, Carbs: 35.2g, Fats: 21,9g

45.   Parsnip Juice

Ingredients:

1 cup of parsnip, sliced

1 large banana, peeled

1 large orange, peeled

1 cup of cauliflower, chopped

A handful of fresh mint, chopped

1 tsp of honey, raw

Preparation:

Wash, peel, and chop the ingredients. Place in a juicer and squeeze.

Transfer to a serving glass and add one teaspoon of raw honey and fresh mint.

Mix well and serve cold.

Nutritional information per serving: Kcal: 336, Protein: 8.5g, Carbs: 103g, Fats: 1.5g

46. Mustard Green and Apple Juice

Ingredients:

1 large green apple, peeled and seeds removed

2 cups of mustard greens, chopped

1 whole leek, chopped

1 cup of Brussel sprouts

1 medium-sized zucchini, peeled

1 cup of parsnip, sliced

Preparation:

Wash and prepare the vegetables. Place in a juicer, one at the time.

Serve immediately.

Nutritional information per serving: Kcal: 284, Protein: 12.3g, Carbs: 83.7g, Fats: 2.4g

47.   Crookneck Juice

Ingredients:

1 cup of crookneck squash, sliced

1 cup of celery, chopped

1 cup of beets, sliced

1 cup of beet greens, chopped

1 cup of pomegranate seeds

1 tbsp of honey

Preparation:

Run the ingredients through a juicer.

Add one tablespoon of honey and serve immediately.

Nutritional information per serving: Kcal: 132, Protein: 6.4g, Carbs: 48.8g, Fats: 1.8g

48. Tomato and Watercress Juice

Ingredients:

5 large tomatoes, peeled

1 cup of watercress, chopped

1 cup of turnip greens, chopped

1 cup of beets, sliced

1 tbsp of coconut sugar

½ cup of pure coconut water, unsweetened

Preparation:

Prepare the ingredients and run through a juicer.

Combine with unsweetened coconut water and add one tablespoon of coconut sugar.

Serve immediately.

Nutritional information per serving: Kcal: 212, Protein: 11.7g, Carbs: 62.7g, Fats: 2.2g

49.   Cantaloupe Juice

Ingredients:

1 cup of cantaloupe, diced

1 cup of baby spinach, torn

1 cup of cranberries

1 cup of parsley, chopped

1 medium-sized cucumber, peeled

1 tbsp of honey, raw

Preparation:

Run the ingredients through a juicer.

Add some raw honey and serve cold

Nutritional information per serving: Kcal: 197, Protein: 10.2g, Carbs: 58.3g, Fats: 2.2g

50. Kiwi and Lime Juice

Ingredients:

1 cup of red leaf lettuce

1 cup of papaya, chopped

1 cup of cabbage, shredded

2 whole kiwis, peeled

1 whole lime, peeled

1 tsp of coconut sugar

½ cup of pure coconut water, unsweetened

Preparation:

Juice the ingredients, one at the time. Combine with coconut water and add coconut sugar.

Mix well and serve cold.

Nutritional information per serving: Kcal: 201, Protein: 7g, Carbs: 61.7g, Fats: 1.7g

51.   Honey Red Pepper Juice

Ingredients:

1 cup of red bell peppers, chopped

1 large red delicious apple, peeled and cored

2 cups of spinach, chopped

1 cup of Brussel sprouts, chopped

1 tsp of honey, raw

Preparation:

Wash and prepare the ingredients. Peel the apple and remove the seeds.

Run through a juicer and add one teaspoon of honey before serving.

Nutritional information per serving: Kcal: 196, Protein: 6.8g, Carbs: 55.6g, Fats: 1.4g

ADDITIONAL TITLES FROM THIS AUTHOR

70 Effective Meal Recipes to Prevent and Solve Being Overweight: Burn Fat Fast by Using Proper Dieting and Smart Nutrition

By

Joe Correa CSN

48 Acne Solving Meal Recipes: The Fast and Natural Path to Fixing Your Acne Problems in Less Than 10 Days!

By

Joe Correa CSN

41 Alzheimer's Preventing Meal Recipes: Reduce or Eliminate Your Alzheimer's Condition in 30 Days or Less!

By

Joe Correa CSN

70 Effective Breast Cancer Meal Recipes: Prevent and Fight Breast Cancer with Smart Nutrition and Powerful Foods

By

Joe Correa CSN

www.ingramcontent.com/pod-product-compliance
Lightning Source LLC
Chambersburg PA
CBHW030252030426
42336CB00009B/357